Autophagy

How to Leverage Your Body's Natural Intelligence to Activate the Anti-Age Process, Detox Your Body and Lose Weight Faster Than Ever Before

GW00686082

Writ

Alaina W. Bolton

Alaina W. Bolton

Disclaimer Notice:

Please note the information contained within this document is for educational and entertainment purposes only. All effort has been executed to present accurate, up to date, and reliable, complete information. No warranties of any kind are declared or implied. Readers acknowledge that the author is not engaging in the rendering of legal, financial, medical or professional advice. The content within this book has been derived from various sources. Please consult a licensed professional before attempting any techniques outlined in this book.

By reading this document, the reader agrees that under no circumstances is the author responsible for any losses, direct or indirect, which are incurred as a result of the use of information contained within this document, including, but not limited to, —

Alaina W. Bolton

errors, omissions, or inaccuracies.

Table of Contents

Chapter 1: Autophagy: Definition and Theory

People have been trying to find the secret of health, beauty, longevity, and weight loss for hundreds of years. If we go back thousands of years into the past, we will rarely see the traces of overweight people, let alone obesity. Moreover, many diseases we know and are trying to fight today did not exist in the past. The lifestyle was significantly different. Moreover, eating habits of our ancestors were much different than ours. In the past, people didn't always have food. They were hunters. Their meals, both the size and the frequency of their meals, depended on their virtue, skills, and luck. Periods of abundance and periods of hunger were interchanging. Even though this does not seem so "healthy" and appealing to a modern man, this is a kind of evolutionary heritage.

Except for several periods of abundance and hedonism through history, our ancestors, both far and recent ones, did not enjoy food the way we do today. Every day or every month to come was more or less uncertain. In the past hundred years, we witness a tremendous increase in severe obesity cases and even deaths caused by obesity around the world. Some regions and countries are the leaders when it comes to obesity, but examples can be found everywhere.

Sedentary way of life, consuming food everywhere, all the time, at any time of the day, eating snacks, eating junk food, no exercising, poor water consumption, and other bad habits we do on daily basis heavily impact not only our weight and physical appearance, but also our overall health, the functioning of our organs, tissues, and cells. As a result, we ourselves significantly affect both the quality and the length of our own life.

At the same time, more and more people are trying to find the right formula that would alleviate the negative effects of our sedentary way of life, slow down the aging process, amortize the effects of stress caused by our hectic lifestyles, and fight various diseases. Some look for the answers in ancient medicine, Ayurveda, acupuncture, natural remedies, and mediation. All of these do have amazing positive effects on our health and wellbeing. However, one natural process stands out thanks to its wide range of effects, effortless implementation, natural origin, and unbelievable benefits. It is called autophagy.

Recently, there has been an increased interest in the term and meaning of autophagy. Most noteworthy, both scientists and common people are interested in their mechanisms, principles, reinforcement, application, and benefits. It seems that everyone now wants to know what autophagy is and how to achieve it.

Although this phenomenon was known much earlier; it was formally discovered, explained, and presented to the world by Japanese scientist - biologist Yoshinori Ohsumi who received the Nobel Prize for Medicine in 2016. It was his research works on autophagy that led him to win the Nobel Prize. Despite its long presence in various medical and scientific texts under various terms, the public became very interested in autophagy only in the past 2 or 3 years.

In this e-book, we will talk about autophagy as the "elixir of youth," a free and effortless means of healthy detoxification and weight loss, and a powerful tool used to alleviate the negative effects of the modern lifestyle, including stress, waste build-up in our body, and obesity. Also, we will try to explain the principles behind autophagy.

Most noteworthy, we will elaborate on the ways of practicing and achieving autophagy and its benefits from various points of view.

This e-book consists of two main parts. The first part, named Autophagy: Definition and Theory, aims to introduce you to the amazing world of autophagy. First of all, we will try to explain what autophagy is in a simple language. Moreover, we will focus on some biological, physiological, and medical terms and processes. This is important as the audience of this e-book may be various regarding background and education. Moreover, we would be very happy if some of our readers would get interested in the topic and try to make further research on autophagy and its principles. The basic medical and scientific terms and explanations we will provide represent a good basis for further research. Similarly, we will introduce you to the past and current research on autophagy. You can look up the references given at the end of the e-book for further reading and information on this topic.

The first part of the e-book consists of several sub-parts. Namely, you can learn more on autophagy through the following sections: What is Autophagy, Types of Autophagy, Autophagy Processes, Autophagy activation processes, Autophagy deactivation processes, and Autophagy Techniques. We will explain what triggers this natural process, what stops it, and we will focus on the most popular method and techniques used to reinforce this process.

The second part of this e-book is called Autophagy Benefits. This part is focused on the ways autophagy affects our cells, tissues, organs, organ systems, and organism as a whole. Moreover, this part of the e-book consists of several sub-parts. They explain each benefit of autophagy separately. In this way, you can jump directly to the section you are interested in, learn more about how it works, and look up your perfect autophagy reinforcement plan. However, we strongly recommend you read the whole book so that you can create a broader image and knowledge on this valuable process. Finally, we will talk about risk groups and who should not practice autophagy techniques and methods without consulting a doctor. In addition, this e-book comes with two appendixes. The first appendix is a simplified 16/8 fasting plan most widely used to trigger autophagy. The second appendix is the autophagy process timeline that can serve you as a guideline of what happens in your body 12, 18, 24, ..., and 72 hours after you start fasting.

We will not discuss the details on autophagy in this introductory part of the book. However, it is important to grasp the essence and a larger image of autophagy at the very beginning so that you can upgrade your information and knowledge in the following sections of the e-book.

Autophagy is a self-healing process, and although a literal translation of the term would not be so pleasant to hear and understand. Namely, it is literally translated as "eating oneself" or "self-eating". We will talk more about the etymology of the word "autophagy" later in this e-book.

This healing process, and above all prevention of various disorders and diseases, is beneficial for the rehabilitation of the whole organism. Simply put, autophagy uses dysfunctional components in our body, which can be cells, parts of cells, etc., transforming them through a kind of a recycling process, i.e. by using accumulated toxins from tissues and cells in order to achieve healing. In this way, the body releases pathological and other waste through the cells that took part in the autophagy process.

In other words, the process of self-detoxification on many different levels in our body takes place through autophagy. Healthy cells recycle the damaged, old, and diseased ones, as well as microorganisms and viruses. By breaking down the "bad" cells, this material is reused for balancing, healing, and protection of one's body, its systems, processes, tissues, etc. Now, let's go into the details and learn more about the science behind this process.

1.1. What is Autophagy? History, research, and theory

Let's begin from the etymology of the word "autophagy". The word itself is derived from the Greek word *"auto"* (self) and *"phagein"* (eating). Therefore, the translation would literally be "eating oneself". It does sound scary at first. Most people have an impression that autophagy is a disorder or a disease when they hear the translation. However, "eating oneself" happens with a higher goal: cleaning oneself.

Basically, autophagy is a mechanism in the human organism by which it gets rid of all "broken" cells (organelles, proteins, dead cells, and cell membranes) when there is no longer enough energy to sustain them. It is a regulated process of decomposing and recycling cellular components in order to clean up the body, protect it from various diseases, heal it, and make it more sustainable and healthier.

In more detail, we can define autophagy as a lysosomal catabolic process of the breakdown of protein aggregates and damaged organelles (Levine and Klionsky 2004) that plays an important role in survival, growth, development, and maintenance of homeostasis (Klionsky 2005).

Today, we can classify and define three different forms of autophagy. Those are defined as chaperone mediated autophagy, micro autophagy, and macroautophagy, differing in physiological function and mode of delivery of the content to lysosomes.

Micro autophagy presents an indiscriminate process in which cytosolic proteins are delivered to the lysosome by invagination of the lysosomal membranes, whereas in chaperone-mediated autophagy molecular chaperones, such as Hsc70, recognize proteins with defined consensus sequence and selectively transmit them to lysosomes. In the process of macroautophagy, small portions of the cytoplasm are packed into a bilayer membrane and thus form an autophagosome. The autophagosome is then fused with the lysosome to form auto-phagolysis in which macromolecular content is degraded by acidic proteases (Mizushima 2007; Yang and Klionsky

2009). The term autophagy is most commonly referred to as macro-autophagy.

In conditions of stress such as starvation, hypoxia, radiation, or cancer cells treatment with various cytostatic drugs, autophagy plays an essential role in removing the damaged intracellular proteins, conserving energy and thus enabling cell survival (Onodera and Ohsumi 2005; Maiuri, Zalckvar et al., 2007; Appel, Herr et al., 2008).

On the other hand, autophagy may also represent a mechanism of cell death in cells with mutant apoptosis genes, during the development of D. melanogaster or in cases where it is inadequate and over-activated (Berry and Baehrecke 2007; Yang, Chee, et al. 2011).

However, the concept "Autophagic cell death" defined on the basis of morphological characteristics is incomplete, according to some scientists, and the presence of autophagosomes in the cytoplasm cannot determine the cytoprotective or cytotoxic role of autophagy in dying cells (Boya, Gonzalez-Polo, et al., 2005).

Accordingly, biochemical and functional conditions upon which we can define the autophagic cell death, i.e. programmed type II cell death, are determined (Gozuacik and Kimchi 2004):

1) Cell death should not be accompanied by apoptosis

2) There is an increase in the autophagic flux of the dying cells

3) Pharmacological and genetic suppression of autophagy saves cells from death (Galluzzi, Vitale et al., 2012).

Autophagy is a process regulated by the products of the ATG gene and can be described by a characteristic sequence of phases: induction of autophagy, creation of autophagosomes (nucleation and elongation), autophagosome maturation, the fusion of autophagosome and lysosomes, and content degradation (Kung, Budina et al., 2011).

Serine threonine kinase Atg1 which is an autophagy-related gene found in yeast and homologs of ULK1 and ULK2 kinase in mammals represent the major molecules that initiate autophagy. During cellular and metabolic stress, the mammalian serine-threonine kinase mTOR target of rapamycin is inhibited. As a result, this allows activation of the ULK kinase within ULK-Atg13-FIP200 complexes and initiation of autophagy. Further ULK kinase by phosphorylation of Ambra1 protein stimulates the translocation of the PI3K complex at endoplasmic reticulum membrane, which is the site of autophagosome formation. Nucleation and elongation of the pre-autophagosome membrane, i.e. the phagophore is controlled by the PI3K complex comprising the phosphoinositide class III kinase (PI3K), serine-threonine kinase p150, Atg14 and beclin-1 (Atg6) protein. In the later process of autophagosome growth and maturation, there are two participating conjugation systems, one composed of Atg12-Atg5-Atg16 proteins, and the other composed of the protease Atg4 and LC3 proteins (microtubule-associated light chain-3).

The LC3 (homolog of Atg8) protein is proteolytically processed by the Atg4 enzyme to form a soluble form called LC3-I. The Atg12-Atg5-Atg16 complex is further conjugated to LC3-I phosphatidyl amine, producing LC3-II that specifically binds to the auto-phagosome membrane. During the maturation process, cytoplasmic contents are packed in a bilayer autophagosome.

When autophagosome formation is complete, it fuses with the lysosome producing an auto phagolysosome in which macromolecular content is digested (Mizushima, Yoshimori et al., 2011; Wirawan, VandenBerghe et al., 2012).

I believe that this is enough biological and scientific data that you might need to understand the autophagy processes, especially if you have a background in medicine, biology, genetics, etc. We will provide more details in the section called "Types of Autophagy".

Now, let's talk about a similar, yet different process taking place in our cells. Namely, another process similar to this one is better known within both the scientific and non-scientific societies. It is called apoptosis and is also known as programmed cell death. What exactly is apoptosis? After a certain number of divisions, the cells are programmed to die. While this may sound creepy at first, understand that this process is essential for maintaining good health. Also, it is very important for the health of your tissues that build up your organs. Consequently, they heavily affect your organs' functions and processes in your whole body. Otherwise, these worn-out cells would gradually deteriorate your overall health and start negatively affecting other cells, tissues, organ systems, and whole organism. You would suffer from premature aging and symptoms, syndromes, and diseases that follow it.

Simply put, cells become old and dysfunctional. Therefore, cell death, along with growth and differentiation, is an essential part of the cell life cycle. Every day, up to 5% of the total body cell number "dies" in the human body. Each person, within one year, produces and breaks down the cell mass that is equal to his/her body weight. This data is simply amazing and makes us suddenly grasp and understand the extent of cell change and replacement that happens in our body on a daily basis. Also, we understand that it is much better to have the cells programmed to die when their "useful lifetime" is over than to remain alive and deteriorate our health. This is the essence of the process of apoptosis, where cells are destined to die after a certain amount of time.

You probably wonder why we are talking about apoptosis. There are common points between these two processes, i.e. apoptosis and autophagy. First of all, they are both classified as programmed cell deaths. They both have a role in renewing our organism and ensuring its proper functioning. However, autophagy is quite different from apoptosis when it comes to several criteria. Let's take a closer look at autophagy and its differences from apoptosis.

Apoptosis belongs to the type I or the so-called "cell suicide". On the other hand, autophagy belongs to the type II. Autophagy is a catabolic process that takes place on a daily basis. It is a routine technique of survival of our body. Our body is designed to attack malignant and dead cells that interfere with the work of healthy cells, eliminating malignant and dead cells from the body, thereby improving the quality of healthy cells that can then function smoothly and maintain the body's health at a high level.

Autophagy is of the utmost importance to our health and is critically important to prevent disease and maintain good health. The main task of autophagy is to collect waste and dispose of it. What is considered waste? Those are viruses, bacteria, accumulations of damaged and dead proteins, cells (organelles), etc.

It is this waste disposal that is extremely important for normal metabolism. I would also mention auto-phagocytosis (another name for autophagy) that is important for the nervous system. The cells communicate with each other via the nervous system. This is important for our growth and development, synapse formation, etc. Nerve cells rely on dynamic cellular processes essential for their proper functioning, whereby they utilize protein synthesis and breakdown, as well as protein quality control in nerve cells as the basis of the nerve cell physiology and pathology.

Why is this so important? Simply put, if there is a disruption of the process of autophagy, which has the role in providing a healthy and clean cellular environment, by creating enzymes and maintaining metabolism, one can suffer from nervous system disorders. How does this occur? Namely, autophagy protects the communication mechanism of cells whose breakdown can cause brain diseases such as dementia and Alzheimer's, as well as cancer. Multiple sclerosis is another field of research related to autophagy. We will talk about this later, in the "Nerve cells" section of this e-book, under the "Autophagy benefits" part.

Moreover, if autophagy works properly, cellular disruption and free radical damage are virtually non-existent or are minimal. Dr. James P. Watson, an expert in molecular biology focused on the mechanisms of aging, said that science now has much more evidence of a link between autophagy activation and longevity than with any other means of promoting longevity, such as antioxidant supplementation, hormone replacement, anti-inflammatory therapies, telomerase activation, or stem cell therapy. These statements reflect the importance of autophagy.

As we have said in the introductory part, autophagy is not a new discovery. Its principles and effects (to a certain extent) were known for more than a few centuries. Namely, another scientist, almost 100 years ago, discovered a way to maximize the autophagy activation. It was Dr. Manfred von Ardenne (January 20, 1907 - May 26, 1997). Von Ardenne was a German researcher, applied physicist, and inventor. He is the owner of approximately 600 patents in the above-mentioned fields, including electron microscopy, medical technology, nuclear technology, plasma physics, and radio and television technology. He found that one mineral, in particular, proteolytic enzymes important for protein metabolism in the mitochondria, regular static strength exercises, and fasting are the most potent activators of autophagy.

The mineral is magnesium chloride, more precisely, magnesium oil that is applied trans-dermally. Magnesium has a strong anti-inflammatory effect and a great ability to increase the capacity of oxygen in the body.

Why is magnesium that important? Most people do not take magnesium seriously when it comes to dealing with cancer and other serious illnesses. Magnesium stabilizes ATP by allowing DNA and RNA transcription and repair. Magnesium deficiency is carcinogenic, and in the case of solid cancer types, a high level of magnesium supplementation blocks carcinogenesis. Magnesium deficiency causes carcinogenesis by increasing the permeability of the cell membrane. The cells then have a smoother surface than normal and have a lower membrane viscosity, analogous to changes in human leukemia cells.

There is a drastic change in the ionic flow from the outer and inner cell membranes (more calcium and sodium, and lower levels of Mg and Potassium). As I already said above, autophagy is a catabolic process by which cells constantly degrade their unnecessary parts in order to stimulate new growth and maintain homeostasis and optimal health.

Now, let's discuss a rather sensitive, yet very important aspect of autophagy. Autophagy balances the synthesis, degradation, and recycling of cellular components for ensuring and allowing better cell function. This is the reason why autophagy, according to some scientists, must be at the very center of the prevention of malignancies (and other diseases).

Conventional medicine focuses on cancer development for gene mutations that attempt to eliminate a series of failed drug therapies, while in reality, damaged DNA is just a symptom of autophagy cessation, which can only be affected by therapies that restore metabolic health.

It is exactly what Dr. Otto Warburg had proven in the 1920s (1923 - 1924). In addition, he won the Nobel Prize for his discovery in 1931. His theory, that cancer is not genetic but a metabolic disease caused by a complete disruption of cellular metabolism was frowned upon by his colleagues. According to Warburg, metabolic mitochondrial disorder, not a genetic predisposition, is the reason why healthy cells suddenly switch to an anaerobic state, taking the oxygen by fermenting glucose where lactic acid is produced as a by-product, the pH drops to 7-6.5, and within 48 hours the cell becomes malignant.

Modern science confirmed this theory many times. Professor Thomas Seyfried from Boston University describes cancer as a metabolic disorder (disease) that changes the entire cell complex, while gene mutations are just one of the side effects that only worsen the body's condition.

Complete DNA sequencing has shown that the mutational signature of certain types of cancer is completely different from one another and even among cells within the same cancer. This nullifies the purpose of the targeted drugs to eliminate the DNA mutation. All this is evidence that a disorder in autophagy activity that leads to complete mitochondrial metabolic disorder is the sole cause of cancer.

In order to further support the autophagy theory and its benefits (which we will address later in this e-book), we will now talk about the so-called mitochondrial theory. It is interesting to think about this question: Why our heart cannot get cancer? What about our neurons?

The mitochondrial theory tells us that our cells alter metabolism through fermentation. Fermentation is the process when sugar ($C_6H_{12}O_6$) in mitochondria is broken down into water (H_2O) and carbon dioxide (CO_2) by multiple gradual processes.

Fermentation processes need to be light and gradual because otherwise, we would develop so much heat in the breakdown process that we would burn out.

Our cells are energy producers that aim to maintain the body temperature of 36.7°C, and each of us has a cooling system that determines what temperature is going to develop in the body. Each of our cells produces 192 J (joules) of energy instead of the maximum 2.814 J, which represents an energy problem in our body, with more variable effects on our body, such as cancer. The most important single effect is the reduced strain on our cell membrane. This reduced cell membrane stress plays a significant role because the cell membrane decides what enters and exits the cell. This altered cell membrane stress causes a lack of oxygen in the cell. At this point, only two options remain for the cell. It may "decide" to die or start life without oxygen, that is, to start consuming more energy than it produces. The by-product of this "decision" is the immortality of the cell. Cancer does not appear because cells divide too quickly, but because old cells do not die.

This anaerobic survival system exists in all our cells. As a matter of fact, the life of an oxygen-free cell is natural, and it implies the ability to produce the energy we need through fermentation in all our cells. Otherwise, we would not be able to survive the first days after conception in the mother's womb. However, there are two places in our body where cancer cannot develop. It is our heart and the neurons in our brain.

Our brain is made up of nerve cells called neurons that cannot be divided, multiplied, and therefore there can be no brain cancer. However, you must have heard of brain cancer many times. We are talking about cancer on the so-called GLIA cells, which are the base of the brain tissue, which does have the ability to multiply throughout life, and that's what they do.

Cells that are the base tissue of the brain are made up of a layer of the mesoderm and encompass most of our brain and are composed of cells such as the glia cells, astrocytes or oligodendrocytes, from which the names of brain cancer types (glioblastoma, astrocytoma, etc.) originate. On the other hand, neuron cells cannot develop   cancer.

When it comes to the heart, its cells are constantly multiplying and the situation is different. Cell membranes have a voltage of -70 mV to -90 mV and as long as this voltage is maintained, it is impossible for the cell to start fermenting, i.e. it cannot become a cancer cell.

The heart undergoes a somewhat higher power output than other cellular structures in our body do, and therefore it is not possible for the cardiac cells to degenerate.

This mitochondrial theory of cancer formation has been deliberately overlooked and neglected for years as if there were no facts that cancer never appears on the heart and nerve cells and that metastases most commonly occur on the liver and lungs, organs whose cells reproduce and divide extremely quickly. Mitochondrial theory completely negates the theory of mutation which the official medicine insists on and bases its methods of treatment.

However, this theory is not yet fully tested and further research on this topic is yet to come. However, the findings we have now are promising and autophagy might be a good way to fight various diseases, including cancer and MS.

Now that we have provided a rather broad and detailed introduction into the amazing width of autophagy effects and benefits, let's get into more technical details regarding the types and mechanisms of the three key autophagy types.

1.1.1. Types of Autophagy

Today, we can differentiate between three main types of autophagy. Those are:

- Micro-autophagy,
- Macro-autophagy,
- Chaperone-mediated   autophagy (Mizushima et al, 2011).

In this section, we want to provide interesting information and findings from different research studies by different renowned scientists around the world who tried to prove the principles and mechanisms behind autophagy in order to understand its benefits and processes. It is important to share this information with our readers, as we believe there will be those with a scientific and medical background. Moreover, anyone interested in autophagy should use these references and information as valuable and trustworthy references for further readings and research.

Different processes and triggers play important roles in different types of autophagy. While in micro-autophagy process, the lysosome membrane invagination occurs, the key in chaperone-mediated autophagy is the role of Hsc70 proteins (Mizushima et al, 2011).

Macro-autophagy, which we mostly refer to when we use the term "autophagy" (in this e-book as well), is the most significant form of autophagy that entails formation of the specific vesicle - autophagosomes around unnecessary and / or damaged proteins and dysfunctional cellular organelles and their consequent degradation by the lysosomal enzymes (Wang and Klionsky, 2011). This process is a form of adaptation that provides energy and allows the cell to survive in a variety of adverse conditions (lack of nutrients, oxidative stress, hypoxia, DNA damage).

Autophagy regulation mechanisms are also very interesting. How is autophagy regulated? Autophagy is regulated by the products of the ATG genes, which stands for autophagy-related genes (Nakatogawa et al, 2009). It can be described by a characteristic sequence of the following phases:

- autophagy induction (depending on the stimulus we distinguish the indiscriminate and selective form of autophagy),
- formation (nucleation and elongation),
- maturation of the autophagosomes,
- autophagosome and lysosome fusion,
- content degradation (Kundu and Thompson, 2008).

The induction phase is characterized by the following processes. In mammalian cells, including human cells, the key role is played by a complex consisting of: homolog Atg1 - ULK (Unc-51-like kinase) 1 or 2, ATG13, RB1CC1 / FIP200 and ATG101 that binds to ATG13 (Ganley et al, 2009). The ULK1 / 2-ATG13-RB1CC1 complex is formed independently of the nutritional status of the cell (Hosokawa et al., 2009). Under nutrient availability conditions, the major intracellular metabolic sensor is MTORC1 (mechanistic target of rapamycin complex 1) phosphorylates ULK1 / 2 and ATG13 and it thus inhibits the induction complex. Nutrient deficiency leads to induction dissociation of the complexes and MTORC1 allowing autophagy induction (Hosokawa et al., 2009).

The nucleation phase relates to the vesicles. Vesicle nucleation involves the formation of phosphatidylinositol (PI) 3-phosphate by complexes comprising: the catalytic subunit of type 3 PI3 kinase (PIK3C3) / VPS34, beclin-1 (BECN1), ATG14, and UVRAG (UV irradiation resistance-associated cancer suppressor gene). A number of proteins are involved in the regulation of autophagosome nucleation. The anti-apoptotic protein BCL2 (B-cell lymphoma 2) binds to BECN1, whereas Rubicon inhibits PIK3C3 activity and thus inhibits autophagy. On the other hand, BNIP 3 (Bcl-2-related BH3-only protein) is a BCL2 inhibitor that in hypoxia states induces autophagy, and this effect is exacerbated by nutrient deficiency (Tracy et al., 2007). AMBRA1 also positively regulates autophagosome formation (Parzych and Klionsky, 2014).

The elongation step requires the activity of two conjugation systems similar to the enzyme complexes involved in ubiquitination. The first system is ATG7, which has the function of an E1 activating enzyme and ATG10, which functions as an E2 conjugating enzyme. These two enzymes allow the covalent binding of ATG12 and ATG5 which, together with ATG16L1, form an E3 ligase-like complex. On the other hand, ATG4 cuts LC3 (which is the microtubule-associated protein light chain) and produces LC3-I. LC3-I then binds to phosphatidylethanolamine via ATG7 and ATG3 and E3 ligases to form LC3-II, which is incorporated into the autophagosome membrane. LC3 and GABARAP (aminobutyric acid receptor-associated protein), which participate in autophagosome maturation, are ATG8 homologs in mammals (Weidberg et al, 2010).

Now that we have provided an insight into the systems, enzymes, and regulation mechanisms behind different types of autophagy, we will talk about autophagy processes, what activates them and what deactivates or stops them, in a more informal, easy to understand language that will help anyone understand how it affects one's body.

1.2. Autophagy Processes

Now, let's go back to the basics. The cells in our body are constantly decaying and recycling their parts, as we have already said. The mechanism behind this process is known as autophagy. Most tissues in our bodies regularly change their cells with the new ones. Each organ needs a certain amount of time to fully regenerate. Also, there are tissues that never change their cells. We have also mentioned this information in the paragraph about the mitochondrial theory. How does this recycling process actually work?

With the help of lysosomes (the organelles responsible for the breakdown of the intracellular material), your body breaks down different protein structures and converts them into amino acids, and later uses those same amino acids to build new cells.

Autophagy

Our body can use its own protein reserves in the form of damaged cells and microorganisms. The average person consumes about 70 grams of protein per day, which is not enough to create the new cells we need. When "protein waste" is used, then our body can receive a sufficient amount of material to recover.

When natural recycling mechanisms cease to function, damaged cells and their components begin to accumulate in the body. The body loses the ability to neutralize cancer cells and infected cells, which can ultimately result in many serious diseases.

Luckily, we can trigger the autophagy process ourselves. There are several different methods. In the following sections, we will learn more about activating and deactivating the autophagy processes.

1.2.1. Autophagy activation processes

Most scientists agree that food and nutrient deprivation is the key activator of autophagy. We all know that healthy and balanced diet is one of the keys to a healthy body and long life. However, you will need to change your point of view here in order to understand how food deprivation, i.e. fasting cleans your body and prolongs your life.

Remember that glucagon is, in a way, the opposite hormone to insulin. If insulin rises, glucagon decreases. Also, vice versa is correct too: if insulin drops, glucagon rises. Normally, as we eat, insulin rises and glucagon goes down.

When we do not eat (when we are fasting, for example) insulin level is low and glucagon level rises. This increase in glucagon stimulates the autophagy process. In this way, programmed and planned fasting, which boosts glucagon, provides the largest known stimulus for autophagy.

This is, essentially, a form of cellular cleansing. The body recognizes old and useless cellular "equipment" and marks it for destruction. It is the accumulation of all this "junk material" that can be responsible for many consequences of aging. Fasting actually has many more benefits than merely being a stimulus for autophagy itself.

Fasting is good for two things:

- By stimulating the autophagy, we clean up all our old, "bad" proteins and cellular parts.

- Fasting also stimulates growth hormone, which tells our body to start producing some powerful new body parts, giving our body a complete rebuild.

You have to get rid of old things before you can put the new ones in. Therefore, the process of cell destruction is just as important as the process of mere cell building or creation. If you simply tried to put in new things in without getting out the old ones, that would be quite difficult. As a result, fasting can reverse the aging process by removing the old cellular junk and replacing it with new, healthy cells.

In order to understand how autophagy processes actually affect our organism, let's take a closer look at what happens in the body when there is a constant supply of food, a steady supply all the time, and what happens during the periods of planned fasting.

When we consume food and during some time after food consumption, digestion and absorption of food take place. During this period, many processes happen and heavily affect our body, both in positive and negative ways. Namely, in response to glucose reaching the bloodstream, the pancreas constantly secretes the hormone insulin, which signals to the cells to use glucose as their primary energy source. In other words, the cells will not use the stored adipose tissue because they do not need it. If we consume food 3 or more times a day, taking more calories than our body actually needs, the fat will not be consumed. On the contrary, the accumulated fat will stay because there is excess energy that the body does not currently need. If the body is constantly digesting new food that you eat, there is no time to deal with detoxification, cell repair mechanisms, and, again, melting the adipose tissue. Adipose tissue is a special kind of fat tissue accumulated in your body that you want to get rid of. However, as soon as you constantly give your body fresh fuel through steady food intake, adipose tissue will stay intact. We will talk more about this type of fat tissue in the Weight loss and Muscle mass sections of the second part of this e-book.

What happens when our body is not digesting food, i.e. when there is no more food to digest? This is when the post-absorption phase takes place. It lasts for 8-12 hours after eating your meal, and only then the body enters the stage of what we call "fasting". When fasting, the body has consumed glucose and a reserve form of glucose, or glycogen, and does not have the need to secrete more insulin (which makes the adipose tissue unavailable for use and degradation). Then, the hormones are released in the body to make the adipose tissue available as the primary source of energy for the cells. Human growth hormone (HGH) is secreted, which not only causes fat to come into a state that makes it easily consumable but also causes muscle tissue build-up or increases. This is exactly what each one of us wants! We want more and better muscles and less fat tissue.

Moreover, noradrenaline secretion also increases in this phase, which also facilitates the fat melting process. Changes in these hormones then lead to an increased metabolic rate. All these factors combined lead to a healthy, natural weight loss that is almost effortless. These are followed by detoxification, proper metabolism, more energy, better sleep, better concentration, as well as long-term benefits, including strengthening the immune system, fighting diseases, improving one's bloodstream, alleviating the aging effects, etc. Shortly, that's how autophagy processes are activated and how they take place in our body. Except this, we will talk about particular autophagy techniques in one of the following sections.

1.2.2. Autophagy deactivation processes

First of all, we want to provide a simple and short answer to this question. The trigger that stops autophagy is – food.

Glucose, insulin (or low glucagon) and proteins all together stop this self-purification and cell recycling processes. Moreover, a very small amount of food at the wrong time is enough to stop autophagy. For example, even a small amount of the amino acid (leucine) can instantly stop the autophagy process.

Therefore, the autophagy process is specific and characteristic for planned and programmed fasting and is something that is not found in simple calorie restriction programs or popular "diets".

Of course, one needs to find the key to a balance. Too much autophagy is not good. Also, no autophagy at all is very bad for your body. This brings us back to what we consider to be the key to everything - the phases of balanced eating and phases of fasting. That's how we, humans, have evolved, that's what we were created for, and we consider it the most natural and sustainable diet for the vast majority of people. We talked about this lifestyle and diet of our ancestors in the introductory part of this e-book. Remember what we've said. Having a steady, constant supply of food is not suitable for our evolutionary heritage. It's not what our body needs all the time.

We cannot constantly be on a diet, nor is it natural. During the periods when we eat, the cells are being built. Then, during the fasting periods, they are being "cleansed". The point of life is in the balance! That's exactly what autophagy is all about, in a simple language and terms.

1.3. Autophagy Techniques

In this section, we will try to answer the following question in detail: How can you trigger and properly practice autophagy?

In his study, Dr. Oshumi used fasting to encourage the body to break down the toxic cells and get rid of the waste. When you fast, your cells live longer and produce more energy. This is the consequence of a proper work of the mitochondria and other cell structures. As a result, there are fewer inflammatory processes in the body. In addition, if you reduce your calorie intake, the level of nitric oxide in your body will increase. What is nitric oxide? It is a molecule that helps us detoxify and rejuvenate the body.

If you practice intermittent fasting by alternating fasting periods with the periods when you eat food, you are helping your body to cleanse itself. Additionally, fasting helps you lose weight and speed up your metabolism. You will have less inflammatory processes in your body and you will strengthen your immune system.

The health benefits of fasting are numerous, including a reduced risk of cardiovascular disease, neurological problems, diabetes, as well as reduced inflammation, oxidative stress, and blood pressure. The best autophagy techniques include various forms of fasting. There are many types of fasting so you can choose the strategy that will best fit your lifestyle.

1.3.1. Types of fasting

- **24-hour fasting**

If you practice this fasting method, you should choose one day a week when you will not eat at all. The fasting period lasts for 24 hours. If you prefer, you can eat your breakfast at 8 in the morning and eat nothing until the next morning at the same time. In the meantime, you can consume various liquids, including water, herbal teas, smoothies, and light soups.

- **16/8 fasting**

16/8 fasting method implies either skipping breakfast by fasting from the previous day until lunch the next day or skipping dinner by fasting from the previous day until lunch the next day or spending 16 hours without food and 8 hours with food.

According to the personal experiences of many people who have tried this method, the 16/8 variant is the simplest one. Also, it is the easiest method to follow; therefore, it is the most popular type of autophagy fasting today. As a result, we will pay special attention to this type of fasting, giving you details about the adaptation period and its benefits.

First of all, remember that you should eat healthy food and have a balanced diet while you are on the 16/8 fasting program. It might sound difficult at first. However, eating healthy food is easy. Once you've prepared the menu and bought the groceries you need, you should get rid of all the "sweet sins" from the fridge. Afterward, everything goes smoothly and your body gets used to this eating program within only a few days.

The advantage of the 16/8 method is that you will sleep during a significant portion of those 16 hours of fasting. It is important to introduce it gradually into your lifestyle over two or three weeks by skipping breakfast or dinner occasionally. In the first week of the "adaptation" period, you should try to schedule food and time on a 12/12 basis. You don't even have to get rid of your favorite foods right away, just choose the healthier versions: yogurt instead of mayonnaise in sauces or coconut oil instead of the regular frying oil. In the second week of the program, for example, you can eat between 10 am and 8 pm which will still provide you a late breakfast, lunch, and dinner, so you will not be starving. During the third week, choose an 8-hour period that fits your daily pace. For example, 10 am to 6 pm or 11 am to 7 pm. During this period, it is recommended to drink plenty of water, as well as herbal teas, and even coffee. Do not try to make up for all the food you have been missing for eight hours: you need to balance the intake of quality, lean meat, eggs, fresh dairy products, fresh vegetables, nuts, and legumes.

After the adaptation period, you can start practicing the full, 16/8 fasting program. Soon afterward, you will start feeling the positive effects as the autophagy process will begin.

- **Intermittent fasting**

If you chose this option, you should eat regularly one day and then fast the next day. This does not mean that you should not eat at all during your fasting days, but instead you should reduce your calorie intake. For example, consume 2,000 calories on regular days and 500 calories on fasting days.

- **Skipping a meal**

If the concept of fasting and autophagy is new and somewhat scary to you, start with skipping meals. Generally, skipping just one meal a day speeds up your metabolism and stimulates the cleansing processes in your body. Remember that you must not eat too much during your next meal after skipping a meal. However, this is not the very best fasting model. It should serve only as a form of adjustment until you start fasting according to one of the regular fasting methods and plans.

- **Limited fasting**

Limited fasting is a type of intermittent fasting. To apply it, you need to eat within eight hours each day. This type is also called "16/8 fasting" because you do not eat for the remaining 16 hours of the day. If this method is new to you, try a less strict schedule. E.g. eat your lunch at 8 in the morning and have your dinner at 6 in the afternoon. In this way, you will spend only 14 hours without food. Once you get used to this, reduce the number of hours you allow yourself to eat.

- **Water fasting**

If you choose to follow this fasting strategy, you must choose one day a week to drink only water or fresh juices without sugar. The best time to practice this type of fasting is spring. However, you can practice it throughout the year.

- **5:2 fasting plan**

5:2 fasting implies fasting two days a week, which do not have to be in a row, and eating regularly during the other 5 days of the week. During the two days of fasting, it is recommended to consume only 500-600 kcal a day.

1.3.2. Other Autophagy Techniques

Even though fasting is the No. 1 autophagy trigger, there are other techniques and methods that will help you activate this process in your body. Those include:

- Keto diet
- Regular exercise
- Olive oil consumption
- Turmeric consumption
- Consumption of coffee
- Lower the intake of carbohydrates
- Sticking to the protein intake prescribed within your 16/8 fasting plan.

Chapter 2: Autophagy Benefits

Autophagy is considered miraculous thanks to its many different benefits. Some potential positive effects of autophagy are currently being researched and tested and are not yet proven. However, the ones we will mention here were proven by scientists in numerous tests, both in vitro and in vivo, on mice and humans.

First of all, we know that autophagy positively affects cellular metabolism. Namely, it triggers detoxification processes. This is the starting point that leads to a series of benefits, including its potent anti-aging effects. Similarly, autophagy can positively affect your weight loss, improve your muscle mass, and condition of your nerve cells. In addition, autophagy has the following positive effects:

- **Autophagy against malign diseases**

Autophagy acts as a preventive and therapeutic agent for malignancies. In recent decades, the rise of malignancies has been shocking the world, so the significance of further research on autophagy and its beneficial effects on cellular health is of the utmost importance. Cancer cells in the process of autophagy are recognized as "excess" cells, i.e. as cells that are unnecessary, and therefore they are decomposed and recycled by our body. This is, currently, the very best way of combating these sick cells without harming the healthy ones. Further research on autophagy and cancer continues.

- **Autophagy against stroke and heart attack**

Autophagy prevents cardiovascular disease and rehabilitates our body during the treatment of such diseases. It is especially valuable in the prevention of heart attack. Namely, autophagy helps maintain homeostasis on a cellular level, and this applies to the cardiovascular system cells too (Schiattarella et al., 2015). Therefore, it will help you reduce and eliminate various heart-related conditions, heart attack, and coronary disease.

- **Autophagy against autoimmune diseases**

Immune system disorders lead to a condition where the immune system itself perceives its cells as something foreign and thus starts self-destruction by producing antibodies. This is how autoimmune processes (diseases) begin. Autophagy will help your immune system with its cleansing mechanisms. Namely, it balances the immune system and thus leads your body towards the healing process. Also, it positively affects the immune response.

- **Autophagy against diabetes**

Hyperinsulinemia, i.e. insulin resistance is a condition in which cells reject normal insulin uptake from the blood that accounts for better flow of energy and functionality in the body. Furthermore, such a disorder leads to excess weight, polycystic ovaries, as well as menstrual cycle disorder that can lead to sterility, etc. In addition, all this further leads to diabetes. During the process of autophagy, the level of insulin in the blood is very low, which activates the hormone glucagon (the one that tends to increase glucose) and then draws all the remaining energy out of the cells, bringing the insulin into balance.

- **Autophagy against bacterial and virus infections**

Autophagy will prevent the onset and development of various viruses, influenza, as well as bacterial infections. It is especially valuable when it comes to typical times of the year when such disease outbreaks occur. Autophagy will definitely help your immune system work much better.

- **Autophagy lowers cholesterol**

The fat accumulated on the blood vessels can be drastically reduced by the process of autophagy. As a result, it leads to an improvement in the general condition of the whole organism.

Also, research has shown that autophagy is an excellent ally in combating dementia, Alzheimer's and Parkinson's disease.

- **Autophagy slows down the aging process**

Reducing calories will also slow down the aging process. Moreover, in addition to nutrition (what, when, and how much we eat), healthy physical activity will help a lot in reinforcing the autophagy effects. Fasting or autophagy will lead to complete regeneration of the organism and thus rejuvenate your cells, tissues, organs, and whole body. When "poor" cells undergo a process of self-destruction, then the process of secreting the growth hormone (which affects the creation of new cells and leads to rejuvenation) is initiated. In addition, the whole life energy for daily functions and processes in your body will increase.

2.1. Detox

Autophagy creates a wheel that is good in getting rid of old parts of cells, can effectively stop cancer growth and metabolic disorders such as obesity and diabetes. The key mechanism it uses to ensure these benefits is detoxification. This is especially important as autophagy is different from other programmed cell death processes as it helps in cases when mere cell replacement is not possible. If cell structures contain "toxins", it is autophagy that heals them. This detox process is not limited only to the cell membrane. It creates a domino effect that cleans your organs, bloodstream, and the whole organism.

There is also considerable evidence that this process controls inflammation and strengthens the immune system. This, in combination with detoxification, has many positive effects on our body and wellbeing.

There are several ways in which one can detoxify his/her organism. Among them, three ways are the strongest and the most efficient. They are easy to apply and the effects are visible within a few weeks.

2.1.1. Three Ways to Autophagy detoxification

We have compiled three ways for you to strengthen your natural autophagy processes that will result in detoxification of your cells, tissues, organs, and your whole body. The first one is to regularly exercise; the second to stay hungry during certain intervals and the last one is to reduce the carbohydrate intake. Let's take a look at the principles behind these autophagy detox techniques.

2.1.1.1. Exercising

If you have ever been exercising intensively, you are familiar with the pain that follows a good training. If the pain you feel afterward doesn't make much sense to you, let's just say that good training stresses your body in a specific, positive way. In fact, training will damage your muscles, i.e. its microstructure, resulting in micro-level stress. This makes the muscles even stronger once they recover and even more resistant to the damage they might face later. Also, sweating helps you get rid of the toxins and waste accumulated in your body both on a micro and macro level.

As a result, regular exercise is actually the most useful method that helps us purify our body without even realizing it. That's exactly why you feel regenerated and refreshed after having good, intense training.

What is the principle behind it? Autophagosomes, the structures formed around the cells that our bodies decided to recycle, are affected by exercise. Namely, the rate of healthy destruction of the cells increases when exercising. In other words, your body will quickly get rid of damaged and dead cells if you regularly exercise. Moreover, the autophagosomes are highly mobile and active in those who exercise, when compared to people who do not exercise.

Daniel Klionsky, a scientist we have already cited in this e-book, works as a cell biologist at the University of Michigan. Moreover, he specialized in autophagy. Klionsky said that it is quite difficult to determine the duration and extent of the exercise required for the onset of autophagy to reach its best level. However, there is no doubt that exercising offers many benefits for your health in general, apart from the possible role of autophagy. Moreover, you should combine different autophagy triggers to achieve the best results.

2.1.1.2. Fasting

Interestingly, most people believe that they can cleanse their bodies if they drink fresh fruit and vegetable juices and eat organic food. There is no doubt that these will provide vitamins and minerals. However, your body needs to occasionally rest from food and drink in order to regenerate and detoxify itself. It must have time and energy to deal with "broken" cell parts and cells, instead of focusing on digesting food all the time.

Although skipping meals is a behavior that is not so good for our organism and that actually increases stress for our body, a regular fasting plan ultimately provides great benefits to our overall health, especially when it comes to detoxification.

Moreover, intermittent fasting has enormous benefits in reducing the risk of developing diabetes and heart disease. In addition, this miraculous feature is directly related to autophagy.

However, there is a great deal of research focusing on whether fasting/interval fasting supports autophagy in the brain. This leads us to the following conclusion: Fasting or intermittent fasting can greatly reduce the risk of developing neurodegenerative diseases such as Alzheimer's and Parkinson's. Detoxification, as a result of autophagy, plays a very important role in these processes.

Also, some studies have revealed that fasting, especially intermittent fasting, improves cognitive functions, brain structures, and neuroplasticity. This means that the brain can learn more easily. However, there is no certainty when it comes to the question of whether autophagy is the main factor in this process as these studies have been conducted on rodents. Since humans are not the same as rodents, it may not always be possible to predict that the results from the studies will be the same as those in humans.

Detoxification through fasting is most easily achieved if you limit your fasting time from 12 to 36 hours. The point here is to drink plenty of water during this time. You can also combine it with exercising depending on your abilities. It can be a light yoga session and some quality stretching movements during your fasting period. Also, you can intensify your training after you finish your fasting and allow your body a few hours to digest the food.

2.1.1.3. Reducing Carbohydrate Intake

As you will learn from this e-book, intermittent fasting is the very best way towards detoxification and triggering autophagy processes. However, this method might be difficult for some people. For example, some people have a metabolism that requires often consumption of small portions of food. Also, some people suffer from certain diseases that can prevent them from practicing the intermittent fasting plan. There are many medical conditions that prevent people from fasting at all.

Therefore, here is another way in which you can achieve similar benefits. All you have to do is leave out refined sugar and sweets. Also, you should stay away from flour and products made from it. In other words, you should reduce carbohydrate intake.

This alternative path is called ketosis. This ketogenic diet is becoming increasingly popular, especially among bodybuilders and those who want to live longer. The main idea is to reduce carbohydrate intake to such a level that the body has to use only fats as a source of energy.

Ketosis allows you to burn your body fat while keeping your muscles in place. Similarly, there is some evidence that suggests that ketosis fights cancer cells, reduces the risk of developing diabetes, and protects the brain, especially against diseases such as epilepsy.

According to scientists, the ketogenic diet is similar to autophagy. Actually, its results are similar to those obtained through the autophagy processes. In other words, by practicing the ketogenic diet, you can see benefits similar to the metabolic changes and benefits of intermittent fasting but without starvation.

Ketogenic diets are very rich in fat: 60% or 70% of a person's total calories should be provided from fat. Nutrients such as peanut butter are very good sources of fat. In this diet, the daily carbohydrate rate is kept below 50 grams.

2.2. Anti-aging

There is a strong connection between autophagy and aging process. Actually, this is one of the reasons why autophagy became so popular in the past few years. Why is autophagy so important in the aging process? Research shows that our aging, that is, the formation of wrinkles and changes in our cells, tissue, muscles, bones, metabolism, and skin over the years, are results of the accumulation of damaged cells that failed to recover.

Let's remind you that autophagy literally means "self-eating", and refers to the body's ability to absorb its own waste and replace poor quality cells. However, like everything else in our body, this process becomes less and less effective over the years. Therefore, not only does our body accumulate more and more waste over time, but it also becomes too slow to clean itself from it.

Aging is inevitable, but controlling 70% of aging symptoms and problems can be affected by controlling the external factors such as diet, pollution, UV exposure, lack of sleep, stress, and sedentary lifestyle. However, the key to success is to optimize the autophagy processes.

Another important thing in the whole anti-aging and autophagy story is the temporary or intermittent fasting. Namely, if you eat constantly, like most of us do, you do not give your cells the opportunity to repair themselves and clean up the waste and toxins that have accumulated. However, occasional short periods of inactivity, i.e. fasting, give them time to take care of the cellular debris.

One should implement a diet plan or fasting plan that suggests that there should be so-called weaker and stronger days. Namely, during the three weak days, one should fast for 16 hours, and eat only for eight hours. If you want to be practical, you can stop eating after dinner, so most of your fasting will last while you sleep.

For example, if you stop eating at 8 pm or even better around 5 pm your first next meal will be around 9 am the next day. Basically, you just skip your breakfast. As long as your fasting period lasts for 16 hours, you can adjust it to the schedule that suits you.

We will talk about a more detailed autophagy fasting plan based on the "weak" and "strong" days in one of the following sections of this e-book.

2.3. Weight Loss

The principle behind autophagy can help you lose weight as well. It's a pretty simple diet and exercise plan that doesn't exclude carbs and fats. The plan is based on the discovery of scientific research for the missing link in the aging process and how to stop it, for which the Japanese biologist Yoshinori Ohsumi won the Nobel Prize in 2016, as we have already mentioned. It consists of thoughtful and balanced nutrition, certain nutritional supplements, and exercise that slow down the aging process or can even help reverse it and ensure a younger look and condition of one's body.

The secret is in the natural bodily process that is the topic of this e-book, called autophagy.

Forget about counting calories, this is the easiest diet ever. Moreover, forget about various tiring and demanding diets, this is the best way to regulate your weight. Moreover, this method that relies on autophagy improves heart health and detoxifies your body.

Autophagy

The process of autophagy, in which cells get rid of their own debris, loses efficiency with aging, and this makes it increasingly difficult for our body to perform cleansing, which causes the accumulation of more and more harmful substances in our organism.

It is also important to note that the constant keeping of our body and cells in the alert mode makes their main task more difficult. In other words, turning the body's autophagy process on and off makes the process of cleansing our bodies more efficient. The same rule can be applied to weight loss. That's why intermittent fasting is one of the best ways to lose weight. We will talk about this in detail later in this e-book.

Earlier scientific studies have shown that autophagy is a response to a stressful situation, which is most easily achieved through high-intensity static exercises (gym training), by taking potent antioxidants, and by alternating between low and high protein intake periods. In addition, all of these three ways can help lose weight. Now, let's learn more about these mechanisms.

Occasional or intermittent fasting is the key activator of autophagy. If we eat constantly, we do not give cells the opportunity to repair and clean up the accumulated waste and toxins.

Short periods of inactivity activate the important enzyme Rpn 13, an enzyme that recognizes (detects) harmful substances in the cell by tagging them with the protein called UBIQITIN, which is a signaling molecule to label old and worn proteins that need to be broken down by a protease.

There is an activation of a group of monooxygenase enzymes (cytochrome P 450) that are potent toxin cleaners in our cells, especially fat cells, which cover as much as 98% of total impurities. Most noteworthy and related to weight loss and overall health, only one kilogram of adipose tissue less prolongs our life by 3 months! Disruption of the Rpn 13 enzyme causes waste to accumulate in our cells and cause disease, especially cancer.

Now, let's learn how to activate autophagy in order to lose weight. Pick three non-consecutive days (e.g. Monday, Wednesday, and Friday, or Tuesday, Thursday, and Saturday) and select them for a restricted diet in which you will fast for 16 hours, eating for only eight hours.

The most ideal way to eat is from 08.00 - 16.00 hours. After that, your fasting period starts and lasts from 16.00 - 08.00. Calorie restriction during the 16-hour temporary fasting period activates autophagy and efficiency is increased by a combination of a protein cycle.

Now, let's learn what a protein cycle is. You consume about 25 grams of protein on the fasting days, and eat larger amounts of protein (50 to 150g) for the remaining four days of the unlimited diet. If you are a total beginner when it comes to calculating calories, let's make your protein intake clearer. For example, 250 grams of white meat (e.g. turkey) yields about 50 grams of protein and one egg about 6 grams of protein.

The protein cycles are extremely important for weight loss, but also play an important role in the anti-aging process. Why is that so? The answer is rather simple. Namely, our body can't make its own proteins, so it's forced to recycle the existing supplies. Low intake of protein promotes autophagy as we enhance the recycling process within our bodies.

It is important to point out the problem with the constant low intake of protein in the form of another symptom of aging, namely the loss of muscle mass responsible for calorie consumption. You definitely don't want to lose muscle mass instead of weight. Also, you don't want to lose your muscle mass as you age. In order to avoid excessive consumption or loss of muscle mass, the body needs to be provided with sufficient protein, and high and low intake cycles help regulate the autophagy process.

It has been proven that protein cycles can be used to reduce the risk of developing diseases such as diabetes, cancer and heart disease. Healthy fats such as olive oil, coconut fat, avocado, butter, nuts, mackerel, sardines, salmon, etc. are extremely helpful too.

When it comes to carbohydrates, you should rely on those with high fiber content such as vegetables, fruits, legumes, and gluten-free cereals. Also, you should consume them later in the day.

This natural metabolic condition is called ketosis and is one of the best ways to promote autophagy. We have already talked about ketosis earlier in the e-book. When we wake up, our bodies are full of ketones. Therefore, in order to get the most out of them, it is advisable to refrain from carbohydrates for at least the first half of the day. To stimulate the autophagy process, minerals such as magnesium chloride and sodium ascorbate are of great use, followed by strong antioxidants such as grape seed extract, E vitamin, CoQ10, etc.

Interestingly, fat is not an enemy in this diet plan. On the contrary, healthy, natural, and unprocessed fats are recommended, especially to start each day with and consume with every meal. Fats have a taste and the more the healthy fats you eat, the less sugar and salt your receptors need for a satisfying feeling when eating food. To start the day, you should have a cup of tea which will awaken the metabolism and keep your feeling of satiety for a long time. Put one bag of green tea or Earl Gray tea with 250 ml to 350 ml of boiling water. You can even combine these two types of teas. Then, add a cinnamon stick into the mixture. After at least three minutes, add a tablespoon of unrefined coconut oil and mix for about 30 seconds with cinnamon. Start with a teaspoon of coconut oil and increase to a tablespoon over several days.

Among other healthy fats, this diet suggests you should consume avocados, butter, nuts, salmon, mackerel, sardines, and organic, quality olive oil.

In this diet plan, even carbohydrates are not the enemy. However, you should be careful when it comes to carbohydrate consumption. You should focus on those with high fiber content such as vegetables, fruits, legumes, and cereals. Consumption timing is also important here. Namely, it is recommended to consume foods rich in carbohydrates later during the day. In fact, when there are no carbohydrates, our body uses fat as fuel. This natural metabolic condition is called ketosis and is one of the best ways to promote autophagy. When we wake up, our bodies are full of ketones, so in order to get the most out of them, it is advisable to restrain yourself from taking carbohydrates for at least the first half of the day.

Foods that are rich in antioxidants, such as dark chocolate and red wine, are also useful for boosting the autophagy process. However, these are recommended in modest amounts.

And what about exercising? You don't have to exaggerate with hours of sports. You should exercise not more than 60 minutes during the days of high protein intake. Exercising plays an important 20% part in the activation of autophagy that cannot be replaced by anything else. Also, you should practice intense interval exercises for two "strong" days and the remaining two "strong" days should be reserved for strength exercises.

Therefore, you should not underestimate any of the autophagy triggers in order to have a full, healthy, and efficient weight loss process.

2.3.1. Inflammations, obesity, and autophagy

Another interesting aspect of autophagy and the way our bodies work interconnects obesity and inflammations. Namely, "low grade" inflammation is a trademark of obesity. Disregarding and omitting this fact are the keys to failure to combat one of the most complex and, at the same time, one of the most poorly understood clinical syndromes. Obesity is an abnormal accumulation of fat and fat cells – adipocytes that are the basic building block of the adipose tissue. However, it is important to know that fat tissue is not just a simple fat storage organ - it is actually an active endocrine organ and a part of the innate immune system that affects many physiological and pathological mechanisms, such as, among other things, glucose homeostasis (steady-state) and inflammation. The endocrine and immunoregulatory role of the adipose tissue is manifested primarily by the activity of the adipocytes themselves but also by macrophages (cells that remove harmful molecules) and which are found in the adipose tissue.

Metabolic overload triggers cellular hypertrophy, an oxidative and inflammatory reaction. Adipocyte hypertrophy also causes cell rupture which triggers an inflammatory response. The release of the inflammatory mediators such as cancer necrosis factor-alpha and interleukin 6 (which is different due to the fact that its main effects take place in different places from its origin) takes place. At the same time, adiponectin production is reduced, thereby predisposing the inflammatory state and oxidative stress. Increased levels of interleukin 6 stimulate the liver to synthesize and secrete a C-reactive protein. Therefore, it is important to know that reliable markers of an emerging disease will be an increase in C reactive protein, but the determination of fibrinogen, plasminogen, PAI-1, ceruloplasmin, and amyloid A will also have a predictive role in determining disease.

Adipocyte enlargement and triglyceride accumulation can be a benign phenomenon - when fat and fat accumulation in liver and muscles is prevented in this way, but inflammation will occur when adipocyte expansion is limited either by impaired adipose tissue development or by impaired fat synthesis. Namely, in this case, the free fatty acids accumulate in the liver and muscles, which will be followed by insulin resistance.

Let's talk about the purpose of inflammation in our body. Inflammation is, usually, an ordered series of events designed to maintain tissue and organ homeostasis. The timely release of the mediators and the expression of the receptors are necessary to complete the program and restore the tissue to its original state. Inflammation has also been implicated as a risk factor for the mechanism of advanced cardiovascular disease, coagulation, atherosclerosis, metabolic syndrome, insulin resistance, and diabetes mellitus. It is also associated with the development of diseases such as psoriasis, depression, cancer, and kidney disease.

Finally, the errors in the approach to addressing obesity are hidden in the fact that they do not affect inflammatory processes because they even tend to be recurrent or chronic in moderate intensity, so the immuno-endocrinological changes in that system start affecting one another by entering a vicious cycle that it keeps repeating itself over and over again.

This is where autophagy can help, both to cure inflammation and obesity. Namely, it positively affects both aspects and conditions. Therefore, it is one of the best ways of breaking the above-mentioned vicious circle.

2.4. Muscle Mass

Nowadays, fasting is not related only to religious beliefs anymore. Many non-religious people practice it. Interestingly, fasting has become a virtually "religious" ritual for them thanks to numerous health benefits.

Still, it is important to know that fasting is not a diet developed by nutritionists and that it excludes certain nutrients, such as carbohydrates and fats. For thousands of years, fasting has allowed humans to survive by working the body in a different metabolic mode during periods of famine.

Today, fasting is a voluntary abstention from food, or food and drink, over a period of time. It can be complete (complete abstinence from eating) or partial (abstaining from only some type of food). Medical fasting can be practiced to detoxify the body. However, it is interesting to observe its effects on muscle mass. First of all, we must know that fasting is not starvation. Actually, it must not be starvation. It is very important to be aware of this. It is not a good idea to drink only tea and water without taking calories at all for longer periods during the day. This, especially low or no protein intake at all, can harm your muscle mass. You might end up losing muscles instead of losing weight.

The body first consumes carbohydrate reserves, which are sufficient for one and a half days. After this period, non-functional or poorly linked cell constituents, so-called cellular waste, become surrounded by a sort of sheath, and enzymes crush those ingredients. Some elements are transported back to the cells and reconstructed by their healthy elements. Autophagy begins within the fasting period itself. However, one can feel the effects after one or two weeks of planned fasting procedures.

In addition, periodic fasting, as well as medical fasting for one to three weeks, lead to a change in metabolic processes.

If fasting takes longer, glycogen (sugar) is consumed and it is needed by the brain. Now, the body starts creating sugar from certain proteins, primarily from the connective tissue. Protein sources are limited because all reserves may not be used up. Therefore, the body now uses fat reserves. Fat is made up of glycerin, which can also produce sugar and fatty acids. Fatty acids are broken down into ketones, which the brain uses instead of sugar to exchange the energy. This is how the internal fat deposits on the abdomen are first broken down. Your metabolism also positively changes. This is very important because over 600 neurotransmitters associated with metabolic disorders such as diabetes; inflammation and cardiovascular disease are produced in these deposits.

Your muscles stay intact during this period. In other words, you will not lose your muscle mass. This is especially true if you practice the protein-rich – protein low fasting regime. This will further strengthen your muscles and prepare them for even larger efforts.

It is also interesting to point out that most people's fat reserves last for weeks. A healthy man, weighing 70 pounds and 170 centimeters tall, can easily fast 40 days according to the intermittent, 16-hour fasting program.

Now, let's talk about the myths and misconceptions. The fears that the muscle (protein) atrophy will occur are largely unfounded. The body has a natural brake, which stores protein reserves in the muscles. Many people who practice fasting claim that their physical fitness has improved and their muscle mass has even increased thanks to fasting. This phenomenon is related to the above-mentioned muscle training thanks to the intervals of high and low protein intake.

2.5. Nerve Cells

Cells communicate with each other through the nervous system. This is important for our growth and development, synapse formation, etc. As we have already mentioned, nerve cells have dynamic cellular processes. These processes must ensure their proper functioning. At the same time, they utilize protein synthesis and breakdown. Also, protein quality control in nerve cells is very important.

Autophagy plays an important role in nerve health too. Namely, if there is a disruption in this process, a healthy and clean cellular environment cannot exist. As a result, this may lead to nerve disorders.

Let's get back to the beginning of the nerve cells story. Cell communication is the essence of the nervous system. Autophagy protects the communication itself. Namely, it protects the mechanism through which the cells communicate and whose breakdown can cause dementia and Alzheimer's.

Most noteworthy, it is interesting to take a look at the autophagy effects in MS patients. While an increased degree of autophagy correlates with (neuro) inflammation, a block in this process contributes to neurodegeneration, which plays a significant role in the pathogenesis of MS. Thus, ATG5 deficiency leads to abnormal intracellular protein accumulation and consequent loss of neurons (Hara et al., 2006). Unfortunately, further detailed data on the role of autophagy in MS is still very scarce. Additional research in this field is being expected.

2.6. Other positive effects of autophagy and fasting

Except for these main benefits, autophagy triggered by fasting leads to additional positive effects and processes in one's body. First of all, a drop in high blood pressure can be observed after two weeks of intermittent fasting. Moreover, the detox processes resulting from autophagy help recover the liver. Most noteworthy, new stem cells are created. This also means that new mitochondria are created. You must know that mitochondria are the energy centers of the cells. These are literally the energy factories within each cell.

Moreover, although fasting in order to trigger autophagy can cause stress at first, after two to three days of the accommodation and adjustment period, one will feel psychically calm, relaxed and balanced. These are consequences of secretion of dopamine and serotonin that work more strongly, so we feel happier and our appetite decreases.

Now, let's take a look at how intermittent fasting affects your cells and hormones. When you are fasting, several important processes take place in your body, both on the cellular and molecular levels. For example, fasting changes hormone levels to make the previously stored body fat more accessible. Growth hormone levels increase, up to 5 times. This contributes to the loss of fat while maintaining muscle mass. Insulin sensitivity improves, and insulin levels drop dramatically, making stored body fat more "consumable". It has been scientifically proven that blood sugar levels can be reduced by three to six percent and insulin by as much as 20 to 30 percent, which is an excellent prevention of type 2 diabetes. In addition to lowering insulin and increasing growth hormone levels, there is an increase in the release of the hormone responsible for fat burning, called noradrenaline. When fasting, the cells begin the process of cellular repair. This includes autophagy, where cells remove old and dysfunctional proteins that build up inside the cells. Changes in the function of genes related to longevity and protection against diseases also occur after a longer period of practicing the intermittent fasting. These changes in hormone levels, cell function, and gene expression are responsible for the health benefits of intermittent fasting and autophagy.

Due to changes in hormone levels, your metabolism can be accelerated by as much as 14 percent. By combining less calorie intake and burning more calories at the same time, this diet triggers weight loss by changing both sides of the calorie equation. According to some studies, weight loss triggered in this way is between three and eight percent over a 3-24-week period, which is actually a significant figure compared to most weight loss studies based on other diets and methods. Most importantly, humans also lose 4 to 7 percent in their waist circumference, indicating that they lose significant amounts of the harmful visceral fats, which are deposited around the internal organs. Furthermore, losing this type of fat can protect blood vessels, heart, and prevent various diseases.

However, keep in mind that the main reason why this type of autophagy works is that you consume fewer calories a day. If you eat enormous amounts of food during the intake period (for example, during the eight hours within the 16/8 fasting method when you do consume food), it is logical that you will not lose any weight.

The impact of fasting on life expectancy and disease prevention is also worth attention and praise. Fasting extends life: if cells have a steady supply of energy from glucose or other nutrients, they are constantly dividing, or "working". As there is a limited amount of partitioning that cells have during their lifespan, they are consumed and died beforehand in conditions of constant feeding, and as a result the organism ages and loses its function. In conditions of starvation, stress occurs, which sends cells the signals that they are supposed to wait for more favorable conditions for division and function, which prolongs the life span of cells and, consequently, our organism.

During fasting, cell repair is also more intense: during the life span of cells, various cellular tissues damage occurs, such as the appearance of the free radicals caused by the oxidative stress. The organism resorts to repair mechanisms only after it has consumed and stored all the food. The process of autophagy is initiated, during which the cell breaks down and gets removed, that is, recycles all the garbage (non-functional proteins) that have accumulated in it over its lifetime, and which it has not been able to throw out of its environment until now. This mechanism protects the cells from toxic build-up, prevents the occurrence of neurodegenerative diseases, slows down aging, and prevents cancer.

Fasting affects genetic expression: there is a change in the function of our genes. Moreover, the genes that cause prolongation of life and protection against disease are expressed.

Weight loss and fat loss are triggered and reinforced through autophagy, as we have already elaborated in the previous sections. With reduced calorie intake and admission to the fat-burning phase, we easily lose weight, and this type of diet is popular among athletes who want to increase muscle mass or simply dissolve fat.

Another role of autophagy is extremely important for human beings. It is its role in immune response and autoimmunity. Autophagy is important for the proper functioning of both innate and adaptive immune responses. At the level of innate immunity, autophagy represents a significant effector mechanism in the defense against intracellular bacteria and viruses (Gutierrez et al., 2004).

The role of autophagy in adaptive immunity is multifaceted. In the thymus epithelial cells, a high constitutive level of autophagy enables CD4 + antigen presentation by T-lymphocytes and clone selection, which is a central mechanism in the emergence of the immune tolerance (Nedjic et al., 2008). Autophagy has also been shown to regulate activation, survival and T-lymphocyte homeostasis (Jia and He, 2011).

More recent studies suggest a role of autophagy in T-lymphocytes affected by other autoimmune diseases. Autophagy exerts a pro-inflammatory effect by leading to apoptosis resistance and hyperactivation of T lymphocytes in patients with rheumatoid arthritis (Van Loosdregt et al., 2016). On the other hand, autophagy suppresses Th9 cells that induce colitis in the mouse and was detected in an increased number in the mucosa of patients with inflammatory bowel disease (Gerlach et al, 2014).

2.7. Potential adverse health effects and risk groups

Like everything in life, what suits one individual may not suit another. In general, intermittent fasting is desirable and has numerous health benefits, but people with special medical conditions should be careful and consult with a doctor or a dietitian before starting their fasting plan.

If you are a person who is lacking nutrients as a consequence of poor nutrition or are a person prone to eating disorders, suffering from diabetes, pregnant or wanting to become pregnant, anemic, a person suffering from low blood pressure or are taking any medication, you definitely need a doctor's permission before starting your intermittent fasting diet.

If you experience any problems during your fasting, stop it immediately.

Ultimately, listen to your body, eat the way that makes you feel the best, don't eat too much food, and choose natural and fresh foods. Moreover, avoid refined carbohydrates and their products. This implies almost all supermarket products. Don't forget to eat various types of food, have a balanced diet, and be moderate in everything!

NOTE: Keep in mind that most of the research has been conducted on animals or has had a small number of human subjects, and larger and further research is definitely needed when it comes to patients with diseases or special medical conditions.

Alaina W. Bolton

APPENDIX 1: 16-HOUR AUTOPHAGY FASTING PLAN BASED ON THE WEAK AND STRONG DAYS

"Weak" days: Monday, Wednesday, Friday

Start your day at 9 AM with a cup of tea. Also, you should have a small breakfast. We recommend half an avocado sprinkled with fresh lemon juice, sea salt, and chili flakes with two teaspoons of avocado oil.

In the evening, at about 5 pm, eat a light dinner, such as Mediterranean chopped salad and asparagus soup. Take up to 25 grams of protein.

Do not exercise.

Drink up to four cups of tea to reduce hunger and boost your mood.

"Strong" days: Tuesday, Thursday, Saturday, Sunday

Have tea in the morning. Exercise up to 45 minutes at a faster pace in the gym. Consume large amounts of protein (45 to 150 g) on average. The fasting starts, preferably, at about 5 pm. It is optimal to fast around 16 hours in order to create the calorie restriction that occurs during temporary fasting, allowing your body to activate autophagy through various channels.

However, to enhance the effectiveness of intermittent fasting, it is suggested to supplement it with a protein cycle. Thus, three days with low protein intake will enhance the autophagy process.

On other days, protein reduction is no longer as effective, so you can increase the amount of protein.

APPENDIX 2:

INTERMITTENT

FASTING TIMELINE

AND STAGES

Being able to track the progress and knowing what happens in your body can be a boost and motivation for your fasting routine. Here's a timeline of autophagy activation and processes in one's body during the intermittent fasting routine.

1ˢᵗ stage: The first stage of autophagy-triggering fasting implies ketosis. This stage starts 12 hours after the beginning of your food abstinence. It is a special type of metabolic condition or state. This is the stage when the body starts to burn the fat. If there is no readily available glucose, our body uses ketones as energy. This especially refers to our brain. As our brain uses ketones, the inflammatory processes decrease and we feel mental clarity.

18 hours after you've started fasting, your body is both producing and using a significant number of ketones for energy. This state is called heavy ketosis. Ketones in the blood can reach 1.0 value, which is significantly more than the regular level. This is the point when ketones start behaving like hormones. Namely, they are sending signals to your body guiding it regarding stress levels and inflammations.

2nd stage: Autophagy is the second stage of fasting. It starts within the first 24 hours after you've started fasting. This is the stage in which your cells start recycling the "broken" and dysfunctional components and cells. Moreover, they are breaking down Alzheimer disease-related proteins. Neurodegenerative diseases are being prevented and malfunctioned segments are being recycled and replaced. In addition, your tissues are being rejuvenated. These processes trigger a circle of beneficial effects for your health.

3rd stage: Growth hormone level rising phase is the third phase of autophagy-triggering fasting program. Namely, 48 hours after you've started fasting, your body experiences low levels of carbs, proteins, and calories. Moreover, its secrets up to five times more growth hormone than before you've started your fasting program. This is related to ketones from the first stage as well. Namely, growth hormone secretion is related to brain activity from the very first fasting phase. In addition, this positively affects your muscles. Growth hormone makes your muscles grow and it also reduces your fat accumulations. The same hormone is responsible for wound healing and for longevity in general.

4th stage: Low insulin levels are characteristic for the 4th stage of autophagy fasting. This stage starts around 54 hours after you've started fasting. At the same time, this increases your body's sensitivity to insulin. As a result, you will experience lots of health benefits, including further activated autophagy process, detoxification, reduced inflammation, less insulin resistance, and increased protection against cancer and other diseases. This is the phase in which your body becomes especially resilient.

5th stage: Rejuvenation of the immune cells are specific for the last, fifth phase of fasting. This stage starts around 72 hours from the beginning of your fasting period. It is characterized by breaking down the immune system cells. Instead of those old, dysfunctional cells, new ones are being put into their place. This results in self-renewal, better immune system, reduced inflammations, better protection against diseases, stress-resistance, and, most noteworthy, regeneration of the blood stem cells. 72 hours after you've started fasting have positive effects on your white blood cells too.

Refeeding: This is the 6th or post-fasting stage that plays an equally important role in the autophagy-triggering fasting process. After a period of low-calorie intake, your body needs to get valuable nutrients. Balanced and nutritious meals are essential for cell quality after the autophagy cleansing process. Moreover, the tissues and muscles need to get enough nutrients. Cellular stress resistance improves in this phase, i.e. after the cells have been repaired and cleaned and they get the necessary nutrients.

The best fasting-eating program includes the 16/8-hour fasting plan. Namely, you should not eat for 16 hours and then you can consume food within the remaining 8 hours. This plan also implies dividing the week into 3 "weak" and 4 "strong" days. The "weak" and "strong" adjectives refer to the protein intake. Namely, you should consume more protein during strong days. Similarly, you should consume less protein during the week days. Also, you should combine your fasting plan with exercising adjusted to your abilities. In this way, the re-feeding phase will have the best effects on your cells, tissues, and the whole organism.

Conclusion

Autophagy is an extremely important natural process for our overall health. It was known for centuries. However, it became very popular after Yoshinori Ohsumi won the Nobel Prize in 2016 for his works on autophagy. This was followed by thorough research in this field. As a result, numerous benefits of autophagy were discovered and proven by scientists around the world. Autophagy became popular and more and more people turn to it both in order to prevent diseases and to cure their existing medical conditions.

Most noteworthy, we now know that autophagy is the crucial segment in disease prevention and maintaining good health. The main task of autophagy is to collect waste from our cells and free our body from it. Autophagy has amazing solutions even when cell replacement is not possible. It performs smart cell recycling processes on damaged cells and removing waste. In this context, waste is dead proteins, damaged and dead cells, malfunction cell membranes, viruses, and bacteria.

Regular cleaning and waste disposal are extremely important for normal metabolism, which is the prerequisite of the proper functioning of other segments and processes in our organism.

As a result, autophagy has numerous positive effects on our wellbeing. Those include detoxification, anti-aging effects, weight loss, improvement of muscle mass and regeneration and improvement of nerve cells, etc. In addition, autophagy prevents and can help prevent diseases such as heart attack and stroke, diabetes, autoimmune and malign diseases, as well as bacterial and virus infections. Also, there is limited research in the field of multiple sclerosis treatment with autophagy. However, further research in this area is necessary.

There are many techniques that trigger the autophagy process. The most effective and efficient one is fasting. Various modes of fasting are used to activate and improve the autophagy process. The most popular one is the 16/8 hour fasting plan. In addition, there are 5:2 fasting programs, water fasting models, intermitted fasting programs, etc.

Apart from fasting, regular exercising and low carbohydrate intake are very good autophagy triggers. Most scientists recommend combining these triggers in order to get the best results.

Processes that follow autophagy include ketosis, heavy ketosis, increase of the growth hormone, detoxification, low insulin levels, and immune cells regeneration.

Autophagy and fasting are usually recommended to anyone not suffering from any disease. Moreover, if you do suffer from a certain disease, you should consult your doctor. Autophagy is useful in treating certain diseases, usually as an additional, supporting therapy. However, you must consult your doctor to make a plan and program of fasting suitable for your health condition.

References

Levine, Y. C., G. K. Li, et al. (2007). "Agonist-modulated regulation of AMP-activated protein kinase (AMPK) in endothelial cells. Evidence for an AMPK -> Rac1 -> Akt -> endothelial nitric-oxide synthase pathway." UJ Biol ChemU 282(28): 20351-20364.

Klionsky, D. J. (2005). "Autophagy." UCurr BiolU 15(8): R282-283.

Mizushima, N. (2007). "Autophagy: process and function." UGenes DevU 21(22): 2861-2873.

Yang, Z. and D. J. Klionsky (2009). "An overview of the molecular mechanism of autophagy." UCurr Top Microbiol ImmunolU 335: 1-32.

Onodera, J., and Y. Ohsumi (2005). "Autophagy is required for maintenance of amino acid levels and protein synthesis under nitrogen starvation." UJ Biol ChemU 280(36): 31582-31586.

Maiuri, M. C., E. Zalckvar, et al. (2007). "Self-eating and self-killing: crosstalk between autophagy and apoptosis." UNat Rev Mol Cell BiolU 8(9): 741-752.

Apel, A., I. Herr, et al. (2008). "Blocked autophagy sensitizes resistant carcinoma cells to radiation therapy." UCancer ResU 68(5): 1485-1494.

Berry, D. L. and E. H. Baehrecke (2007).
"Growth arrest and autophagy are required
for salivary gland cell degradation in
Drosophila." UCellU 131(6): 1137-1148.

Yang, Z. J., C. E. Chee, et al. (2011). "The
role of autophagy in cancer: therapeutic
implications." UMol Cancer TherU 10(9):
1533-1541.

Boya, P., R. A. Gonzalez-Polo, et al. (2005).
"Inhibition of macroautophagy triggers
apoptosis." UMol Cell BiolU 25(3): 1025-
1040.

Gozuacik, D. and A. Kimchi (2004).
"Autophagy as a cell death and tumor
suppressor mechanism." UOncogeneU
23(16): 2891-2906.

Galluzzi, L., I. Vitale, et al. (2012). "Molecular definitions of cell death subroutines: recommendations of the Nomenclature Committee on Cell Death 2012." UCell Death DifferU 19(1): 107-120.

Kung, C. P., A. Budina, et al. (2011). "Autophagy in tumor suppression and cancer therapy." UCrit Rev Eukaryot Gene ExprU 21(1): 71-100.

Mizushima, N., T. Yoshimori, et al. (2011). "The role of Atg proteins in autophagosome formation." UAnnu Rev Cell Dev BiolU 27: 107-132.

Wirawan, E., T. Vanden Berghe, et al. (2012). "Autophagy: for better or for worse." UCell ResU 22(1): 43-61.

Mizushima N, Komatsu M, 2011.
Autophagy: renovation of cells and tissues.
Cell 147, 728-741. [PubMed]

Wang K, Klionsky DJ, 2011. Mitochondria
removal by autophagy. Autophagy 7, 297-
300. [PubMed]

Nakatogawa H, Suzuki K, Kamada Y,
Ohsumi Y, 2009. Dynamics and diversity in
autophagy mechanisms: lessons from yeast.
Nature reviews Molecular cell biology 10,
458-467. [PubMed]

Kundu M, Thompson CB, 2008. Autophagy:
basic principles and relevance to disease.
Annual review of pathology 3, 427-455.
[PubMed]

Ganley IG, Lam du H, Wang J, Ding X, Chen S, Jiang X, 2009. ULK1.ATG13.FIP200 complex mediates mTOR signaling and is essential for autophagy. The Journal of biological chemistry 284, 12297-12305. [PubMed]

Hosokawa N, Hara T, Kaizuka T, Kishi C, Takamura A, Miura Y, Iemura S, Natsume T, Takehana K, Yamada N et al, 2009. Nutrient-dependent mTORC1 association with the ULK1-Atg13-FIP200 complex required for autophagy. Molecular biology of the cell 20, 1981-1991. [PubMed]

Tracy K, Dibling BC, Spike BT, Knabb JR, Schumacker P, Macleod KF, 2007. BNIP3 is an RB/E2F target gene required for hypoxia-induced autophagy. Molecular and cellular biology 27, 6229-6242. [PubMed]

Parzych KR, Klionsky DJ, 2014. An overview of autophagy: morphology, mechanism, and regulation. Antioxidants & redox signaling 20, 460-473. [PubMed]

Weidberg H, Shvets E, Shpilka T, Shimron F, Shinder V, Elazar Z, 2010. LC3 and GATE16/GABARAP subfamilies are both essential yet act differently in autophagosome biogenesis. The EMBO journal 29, 1792-1802. [PubMed]

Schiattarella GG, Hill JA. Therapeutic targeting of autophagy in cardiovascular disease. *J Mol Cell Cardiol.* 2016 Jun;95:86-93. DOI: 10.1016/j.yjmcc.2015.11.019. Epub 2015

Nov 18. PubMed PMID: 26602750;
PubMed Central PMCID: PMC4871782.

Gutierrez MG, Master SS, Singh SB, Taylor
GA, Colombo MI, Deretic V, 2004.
Autophagy is a defense mechanism
inhibiting BCG and Mycobacterium
tuberculosis survival in infected
macrophages. Cell 119, 753-766. [PubMed]

Nedjic J, Aichinger M, Emmerich J,
Mizushima N, Klein L, 2008. Autophagy in
thymic epithelium shapes the T-cell
repertoire and is essential for tolerance.
Nature 455, 396-400. [PubMed]

Jia W, He YW, 2011. Temporal regulation of
intracellular organelle homeostasis in T
lymphocytes by autophagy. Journal of

immunology (Baltimore, Md: 1950) 186, 5313- 5322. [PubMed]

van Loosdregt J, Rossetti M, Spreafico R, Moshref M, Olmer M, Williams GW, Kumar P, Copeland D, Pischel K, Lotz M et al, 2016. Increased autophagy in CD4(+) T cells of rheumatoid arthritis patients results in T-cell hyperactivation and apoptosis resistance. European journal of immunology 46, 2862-2870. [PubMed]

Hara T, Nakamura K, Matsui M, Yamamoto A, Nakahara Y, Suzuki-Migishima R, Yokoyama M, Mishima K, Saito I, Okano H et al, 2006. Suppression of basal autophagy in neural cells causes neurodegenerative disease in mice. Nature 441, 885-889. [PubMed]

Printed in Great Britain
by Amazon